"...Wonderful book. Highly recommended for anyone struggling to conceive and their friends, family, and support network."
-Serena H. Chen, MD

"...Laughing IS Conceivable is like a breath of fresh air..."
-Alice D. Domar, PhD

"...A 'must read' for all patients, partners and family members."
-Richard P. Marrs, MD

"Humor uplifts us in the most challenging of times. Thanks to Lori for sharing many laughs."
-Robert J. Kiltz MD, FACOG

"Hilarious! Highly recommended to anyone who needs a good laugh as they go through infertility treatments."
-Eve Feinberg, MD

"I wish every Reproductive Endocrinologist would include Lori's book in their treatment protocol."
-Lisa Rosenthal, Patient Advocate-RESOLVE New England Board Member

"...Wonderfully light-hearted and entertaining way of discussing a serious, sensitive, and frustrating subject."
-Laurence A. Jacobs, MD, FACOG

The above excerpts are from: "Wh   ᵀ   ᴬ   Saying About Laughing IS Conceivable" p. 105

D1014033

Laughing *IS* Conceivable

Other Books by the Author

Laughing *IS* Conceivable No Matter How Many You're Carrying: Insanity in its Infancy

Laughing *IS* Conceivable: From End of School to Back-to-School (I Love my kids. I love my kids. I LOVE MY KIDS!)

La Risa *ES* Concebible: Una Mirada Extremadamente Graciosa de Una Mujer, al Mundo Extremadamente No Gracioso de la Infertilidad.

Laughing *IS* Conceivable:

One woman's extremely funny peek into
the extremely unfunny world of infertility

by Lori Shandle-Fox

LAF Publications

ISBN 978-0-692-95011-1 (paperback)

Front Cover Design: Adrienne Michalski
Front Cover Photo: Hilary Pearce
Cover Model: Heather Wilson
Back Cover Design: Sandy Vazan

I dedicate this book:

To my four true loves: Lloyd, Jacob, Carly and Hayley. Thank you for filling my life with joy, inspiration, and humor.

To my wonderful parents, Jerome (Jerry) and Harriet Shandle who have always brought love and laughter into my life and haven't let a little thing like death come between us.

Table of Contents

Foreword by Sanford M. Rosenberg, M.D..ix

Acknowledgements xiii

Introduction...xv

Chapter 1: "Loss of Mind: The Only Guaranteed Side Effect"...................1

Chapter 2: "The Husband: What's *He* Got To Do With It?" 11

Chapter 3: "It's All in the Wrist" aka 'I Know What YOU Just Did!'"....21

Chapter 4: "The Taming of the Yentas".......................................30

Chapter 5: "Be Nice to the Office Staff or They'll Spit in Your Eggs"......42

Chapter 6: "Waiting Room Games"...55

Chapter 7: "OOOOOOh Mr. Grant"...70

Chapter 8: "Will the Months and Months of Madness (N)Ever End?.......85

About the Author...103

What the Experts are Saying About Laughing IS Conceivable...............105

Foreword by Sanford M. Rosenberg, M.D.

I began my Fellowship in Reproductive Endocrinology on the day in 1978 that Louise Brown, the first baby born as a result of *in vitro* fertilization, was introduced to the world, indelibly date-stamping my personal career in infertility care as having taken place completely in the IVF era. It has been a rollicking ride, especially in the early days.

I performed the first IVF in central Virginia, in 1986, but it seemed a little like asking patients to buy a lottery ticket: "Ya wanna try IVF? It's never worked for anyone else, but *maybe* it will for you!" We were desperate to get someone pregnant, but always, even after our first few successes started creeping in, we *always* talked about IVF as the *dead last* thing we had to offer, never really up front, in the beginning of treatment, because it was just too infrequently successful to be a viable first option.

I recall a conversation with a colleague of mine in the early days, after we had been to a series of scientific sessions on IVF with presenters who may have started IVF perhaps two months before me, and each discussing his own ideas of what particular "black magic" they used. He said, in a tired and somewhat frustrated voice, "Do you think this will ever be 'routine'?" I knew he meant could we ever get to the point where we could just suggest IVF to a couple and actually *expect* that they would get pregnant?

Over the years, I have recalled that conversation many times- when our success rates stalled at around 20%, when we were regularly getting about 1 in 3 patients pregnant, when we first had a year at 50%, and now when success rates above 50% per attempt in young women are commonplace. I am grateful to have been a part of that "pioneering" evolution. Granted, we do not achieve 100% success rates, but just to be able to meet a new couple for the first time and say: "You really need to do IVF" and know I can very likely fulfill their desire for a baby (to quote Dustin Hoffman in *Little Big Man*), "makes my heart sing".

There are, of course, other and less complex infertility treatments that are very appropriate for many couples, and other ART (assisted reproductive technology) treatments besides IVF, like intrauterine insemination and ovulation induction, but it is so satisfying that I am at a point in my career—and IVF in its evolution—that IVF is often my ace in the hole that I can pull out if all else fails.

No matter how good we get at treatment, however, all Reproductive Endocrinologists need to remember that at the core, there is an anxious, frustrated, and often even "hostile" patient/couple who is often at their wits' end. They've been "through the mill", figuratively (and sometimes literally). They are fragile, often teary, and usually overwhelmed by the time we see them. I frequently tell my staff that these initially "hostile" patients are not really angry at *us*- we've had no opportunity yet to make them mad- but they are mad at the world and frustrated by the situation in which they find themselves, and we need to understand that. Sometimes laughter and levity work. Sometimes it's the hundreds and hundreds of baby (and big kids' and teenagers') pictures on our "Success Wall" that does it. But mostly it's a whole lot of TLC and the belief that someone cares and understands and will go to the wall for them that reassures them and gives them hope.

I understand their frustrations well. My wife and I spent many years on the patients' side of the desk before our first was born and we know the trauma of a temperature 1/10 degree lower than you thought it "should" be or the loss of control you experience when someone tells you when you "should" have sex and worse, when you shouldn't. You get to the point where you forget that you used to have sex because you enjoyed it, and not because it was the "right" day. And there's that worst menses of all, the one that comes a day or two late, the one you were sure wasn't coming this time, but it did anyway. These are all terribly painful, and frequently unavoidable, but by no means rare or even uncommon.

Lori Shandle-Fox has written a great book that captures these moments of supreme frustration. She somehow brings smiles, chuckles, and even belly laughs to the people who understand only too well just what pain she has experienced and how she can teach them to endure this adversity with a sense of humor and a sense of belonging- of not being alone. I commend her for her efforts, and will encourage my patients to read it.

Sanford M. Rosenberg, M.D.
Richmond Center for Fertility and Endocrinology-
Richmond, Virginia

Acknowledgements

To DC Stanfa, Dr. Sanford Rosenberg, and Dr. Bobby Webster: Three people who barely know me from the proverbial hole-in-the-wall who have moved me (and this book, literally) with their boundless generosity.

To fertility clinic nurses everywhere: You are the front line for, and in the tight trenches with, every infertility patient and his/her attitude, anger, frustration, fears, and tears. Whatever you're getting paid, for 99% of you, it ain't nearly enough.

Laughing _IS_ Conceivable: The Introduction

Infertility. There I've said it. And I can almost guarantee you that I'm never going to say it again in the next however many thousands of pages. I'll also try avoiding the letters IVF in sequence. We all know they stand for "Isn't Very Fair". So I'm going to kvetch about this whole business right here in this intro and then move on. If you're embroiled or about to be embroiled in this journey, you don't need another book, friend, or professional telling you about statistics, syringes, doing it standing up, or drinking green tea while doing it standing up. You need... a lot... to laugh... a lot.

So this is what you and I already know and what I want you to forget for at least the time it takes you to read this book:

Why IVF does indeed stand for:

"Isn't Very Fair":

1. Maury Povich's show gives DNA tests to five or ten guys at a time so one woman can find out who fathered her baby. I've had a monogamous relationship for years and I can't conceive.

2. Every day, I see parents screaming at or smacking their children who are barely old enough to walk. I would be a loving parent.

3. If you watch *Judge Judy*, you know that alcoholics and drug addicts seem to have no trouble conceiving. I don't drink at all. I eat well and exercise.

4. Three women I work with are pregnant. None of them was really planning to be. They just got lax with the birth control. I've been trying for two years.

5. Women have seven kids by seven different fathers: All of whom are in jail. My taxes are paying for their kids...as if the twenty thousand dollars for my treatment wasn't enough.

The following lines are for you to add some of your own favorite conception complaints about society as a whole or your friends and neighbors in particular.

_____

_____

_____

_____

And this, mostly ladies and a few brave gentlemen, officially closes the vents on our kvetch and gripe segment. Now, rip out this miserable, whiny page and tear it to smithereens. I'm serious. I don't want its negative energy to infect the rest of the book. (If you're reading this in the e-book version, well, just keep your finger a'movin' and never look back.)

And let me say right here: I'm truly sorry you have to go through this. I'm also truly sorry I hadn't met and married my husband ten years earlier so my eggs would have been ten years younger the first day I tried to get pregnant. But that doesn't make any difference right now. The only thing that does matter right now is this: We're all doing or about to do everything we can medically to create children. Obsessive worrying and good ol' fashioned freaking out, while hard to avoid and often temporarily satisfying, are not medically required and could potentially end up doing more harm than good. So here's a chance to take a break and hopefully laugh your butt off before it's time to jam another needleful of progesterone into it.

Are there studies linking fertility treatments and early senility? One night as I undressed, I caught myself in the mirror. It appeared, I had not only shaved only one leg that morning, but I apparently had been wearing my underwear inside out the entire day. I shared my idiocies with my husband as I slipped into bed and turned out the light. We both attributed my mental demise to the hormones. Then I saw something. Besides sensing my husband still smirking in the dark behind my back, I saw something: A light coming from somewhere in the house. I got out of bed to investigate, returning a moment later.

"What was it?" he asked, still smirking in the dark I'm sure.

"You left the freezer door open." I responded.

So maybe it's the hormones...or maybe it's something else.

Laughing *IS* Conceivable: Chapter One

"Loss of Mind: The Only Guaranteed Side Effect"

"We've been trying to have a baby for five years and we went to this facility and it's like a million dollars and we've been doing this procedure for months and months and I was sure it worked, then it didn't and I have to go there twice a week and then I have to go to work afterwards. And my husband comes with me but then he has to take two buses and a train to get back to work and he's starting to hate me and I really hate needles and I'm on three medications that I probably mixed up last night and the insurance isn't covering any of it and my mother-in-law wants to know why I'm not pregnant yet when her neighbor's daughter who got married a week after I did already has three kids." And with this insanity brunching on our minds, we head down the Hormonal Highway straight for Paranoia Park.

Underwear It Counts

I've become my own crotch watcher. From the time I decided to try to conceive naturally throughout this whole process, I've been staring at my panties. I'm serious. I rarely take my eyes off of them.

"Am I getting a period? I hope not. That means I'm not pregnant."

"Am I getting a period? I hope so. That means the drugs are clearing out of my system and everything's getting back to normal."

"Am I getting a period? I hope so. That means I start my blood tests tomorrow and I can try again."

"Am I getting a period? Is that a spot or just underwear lint?"

"Am I getting a period? I think I smell something! Maybe it's fabric softener."

"Am I getting a period?! Or is that just a reflection from my tights?"

"Am I getting a period?! I think I hear it coming!"

"Am I getting a period?! Are these milkshake cramps or menstrual cramps?!"

The Insanity Flows

Once I've determined that my signs and symptoms definitely equal the onset of my period, I must embark upon a new psychosis.

I know that I must get my blood and uterine lining checked on day two of my cycle. But do I really know what day two is? Three days ago I felt bloated. Was that day one? Two days ago I got achy. Was that day one? Yesterday I saw some discoloration. Not quite "the beginning", more the "on-the-way". Was *that* day one? Then today I got it at night. So is today day one and tomorrow day two? Or is today day nothing and tomorrow day one because it's the first full day? And if I was in the Middle East, they go by a lunar or lunisolar calendar and their days start at sundown the night before. And if this was leap year it probably wouldn't matter. But if I got it on leap day, would I start counting from February 29th or March 1st?

A nurse told me last Friday that I should start counting the first day of my normal downpour. Not inclement weather. Not mild precipitation. Not intermittent showers. It would have eased what's left of my mind if she'd told me two years ago when I began the procedures. Maybe I should have asked her two years ago.

Other Unendorsed Reality Checks aka:
"Why Nurses Have Voicemail"

"I know the nurse said to take 250 iu of the Follistim tonight. I clearly remember that's what she said. I wrote it down right here. Look '250'. I'd better call her and make sure."

"The nurse said to dial the Follistim pen until the dot is in the middle of the '250' mark. But it doesn't stop in the middle middle. Should I use the top middle or the bottom middle of the dot? Should I switch off? One night the top middle and the next night the bottom middle? I'd better call her and make sure."

"I know that I must keep the Follistim refrigerated at all times. But it took a half hour on the unrefrigerated train from the pharmacy to my kitchen. Truth be told, it was more like thirty-six minutes. Maybe it fell below medically acceptable temperature standards. Maybe it's garbage now. I did everything I could. I begged the conductor to skip stops. I nonchalantly pressed my drug bag against the cold soda the guy next to me was drinking and offered to pay his dry cleaning bill. But there were still those thirty-six to fifty-one minutes! Will I have to throw out the whole batch of drugs and rent an apartment closer to the pharmacy? I'd better call the nurse and make sure."

My husband had accompanied me on this little pleasure tour. At one point during the merry voyage he said: "I believe this is your stop." I squinted out the window through the sparkling sunshine to see Creedmoor: A famous mental institution.

Needling at Night

My neuroses seem to flourish most after dark- almost always after office hours. At 9:00 one evening, my husband and I were clustered over the bathroom sink examining syringes.

"I could swear last time the needle wasn't this thick." I was certain.

"It's the same needle." He insisted in monotone.

"What if it's not? What if I puncture my spleen? I have to get up for work at 6 a.m. I don't have time for a punctured spleen. And after all the time and money we spent? They probably won't let me go through with the retrieval until I get my spleen fixed. And how much is THAT going to cost?!"

His mouth gently suggested I have the answering service page whomever was on call. His eyes, however, told a more sinister tale. Clearly he was mentally rehearsing how he would explain the syringe in my neck to the cops who clamored into my bathroom in response to his "frantic" 911 call.

As there was nearly a full one-tenth of one percent chance that I was about to use the wrong needle, I took his back-handed suggestion and had the answering service page Dr. Martin who was on call for emergencies.

Ten minutes later, Dr. Martin called me back with party noise in the background. Counting my husband and the answering service guy, Dr. Martin was the third male to hate my guts within the quarter hour.

"What IS it Mrs. Fox?"

I explained about my spleen and the police taking down the report of my "accidental" death. He was very understanding:

"It's the right needle. Stick it in your behind and go to bed!" Click.

I turned to my husband, phone in one hand, syringe in the other.

"He didn't mean I should leave it in all night did he? I don't remember EVER doing that before."

Leaning up against the bathroom door frame, he looked at me, murder still in his eyes: "Why don't you page him again and ask?"

I pictured the two of them buddying up at the inquest.

Dr. Martin: "Look, I'll say you were with *me* all evening…"

Dr. Sanford Rosenberg wrote something in the foreword about fertility treatments taking the romance and spontaneity out of the bedroom because you're told "when to have sex and when not to." I admire and respect Dr. Rosenberg greatly, but to this statement I can't relate. I recall vividly one night in particular, months before ever having set foot into a fertility clinic. At circa 10:30 that evening, I boldly ventured over to my husband's side of the bed for a second time. As I made the one foot trek, I flung my arm over him and tried to roll him towards me. (Have you ever moved a tree stump out of the roadway?) While I gazed longingly into his shoulder blade, he muttered: "It's late. Don't be greedy."

Laughing *IS* Conceivable: Chapter Two

"The Husband: What's *He* Got To Do With It?"

Often I will refer to "the husband". It may not be politically correct or accurate in your case because you may have a boyfriend, significant other, life partner, chum, donor, willing participant, or friendly neighborhood ejaculator. So please don't get offended if sometimes I use "husband" as an include-all title. I just think it sounds nicer than "the guy with the plastic cup". In college, I had a friend who always introduced her male companion as her "lover". Finally one day, after having witnessed dozens of partygoers squirm at this introduction, I suggested to her:

"Carmen, why don't you just say: 'This is John, the guy that I do?'"

My husband has been a tremendous help and comfort to me all of these months. Thank goodness.

Because there are times in life when the inequities in the world between men and women are blatant. Never are they more so than during this process. Any woman who's ever been pregnant must feel the same. I imagine she's gotten the joy of having leg cramps, losing more than one lunch, constipation, and excruciating back pain while he's experienced the agony of having to replace wild touchy-feely with bowling. The women's movement has made some great strides but when are we going to march with this sign: "Gonal-F for Men! Gonal-F for Men!"?

I realized the scales were quite tipped very early on. My husband and I were on equal footing, or equal examining tables for the first week. He had blood tests. I had blood tests. He gave a sperm sample. I took some hupahepahickagram to make sure my fallopian tubes hadn't closed down for construction as a result of rough sixth grade dodge ball. So basically, he got to fancy himself as the bologna in an Olsen twin sandwich and I got to hold my urine for several hours. And the road to equality begins to fork.

He's declared to be fine. Even though my husband swims above water like an elderly lady in the ocean at Atlantic City, his sperm are all somehow close relatives of Mark Spitz. (If your fertility issues aren't age-related as mine probably are, pretend I said "Michael Phelps", will ya?) His sperm are fast, straight, and plentiful. They're Mensa material, have a wry sense of humor, speak fluent Aramaic, and understand Tom Stoppard. I had to squeeze my husband's head until it popped so we could get through the exit to the doctor's office. Since then, his participation has been pretty much relegated to reading in the waiting room and picking up prescriptions.

I, on the other hand, felt like I had signed on for some perverse reality show. "Eat a scorpion? Ha! Try taking a Medrol without a cracker! Get that taste in your mouth! Do it! Do it!" Who knew what I was getting into?

"Okay so you're going to come in on the second day of your period and we'll take this stick that has a condom with lubricant on it and put it up there to check your lining and then you'll take this pen and put a cartridge in it (it's really easy) and dial it to two hundred and then pinch the fleshy part of your stomach and jam it in." I was like: "What? Are you guys making this up as you go? Wait. I'm supposed to do whateverything you just said at home? Are you serious? My degree is in Spanish."

Luckily, unlike a reality show, all of us women don't have to live together for the duration of our treatments. It would be like an old black and white

Charlie Chan movie. It would be a dark and stormy night. The lights would go out, and when they came back on, all of us would be dead on the parlor floor with Follistim pens sticking out between our shoulder blades. Autopsies would be conducted to find the murderess/suicideress: The woman in the throes of the worst mood swing at the time of death. A new group of contestants would have to be brought in every three days.

At any given moment, there's a great chance that I would be the one determined to be in the throes of the worst mood swing. And if you combine my pendulum trip with being fed up with shots and ultrasounds and pills and my husband's face and blood tests and my husband's face, and doctors' faces and nurses' faces and technicians' faces, and my husband's face, I usually say something loving and considerate to my husband like: "What do YOU know about it? All YOU have to do is jab me in the ass and touch yourself inappropriately!"

As for the former of his two responsibilities: For the past several months, I've been Googling mercilessly. I'm convinced that this whole nightly progesterone shooting up ritual isn't necessary. I truly believe that it's part of some sadistic plot jointly concocted by doctors and husbands to get back at us for our many, shall I say, inadvertent bouts of insensitivity directed at them. So while I've been frantically typing in the search field: "Progesterone+Husband+Conspiracy" and asking WebMD questions like: "How many needle points can you get into the average North American butt cheek?", my husband is having a ball!

I monitor him in the medicine cabinet mirror. I want to know what's going on back there at all times. The first time or two, I could tell he was nervous.

He'd bite his lip and his eyes would shift. Where did the upper outer quadrant end? Had the ice frozen the spot sufficiently? Would the long needle still cause great pain? Then, after a couple of days, I noticed a distinct change in his demeanor through the looking glass. His eyes were fixed. His tongue hung out. He had a demonic look in his eyes and a Cheshire cat smile. He was enjoying it! I could read his mind. Days ago it was saying: "Oooh. This has got to hurt." Now he was thinking: "There! Take that!"

As the weeks passed, the face in the mirror softened. He took longer back there. His eyes displayed the concentration of an artist at work. After he finished one evening, with great difficulty and the help of two hand mirrors, I manipulated myself around. I had to see his handiwork. Sure enough, there it was, plain as day: The evening sky.

Each night he had painstakingly added one

star of a constellation. The left cheek had apparently begun with the North Star and grown into Ursa Minor. Then, with growing confidence, he had gotten bold. The right cheek had what resembled Cassiopeia, The Lady in the Rocking Chair, and two-thirds of Orion. See, everything happens for a reason. If I'd never had problems conceiving, my husband may have gone his entire life without knowing he had this enormous talent for Ass-tronomy.

I admit that I've definitely relaxed during the nightly dose of progesterone also. At first, we were both panicky doing this whole ice your butt, draw the oil from the vial, inject the one and a half inch needle deal. Now it's routine. We used to hover over the bathroom sink making sure everything was laid out properly: Alcohol pad (check), syringe (check), progesterone vial (check), ice (check). Now he just jabs me in the living room while we're watching

Jeopardy! "What is...... Macedonia? Oh, you did it already?" This whole thing has turned us into swinging hippies. Hey man, look at us! We're dropping drawers and shooting up in the living room...with the shades up! We're practically nudists!

And we're getting more brazen by the minute. I'm afraid at Thanksgiving, my husband might stand up at dinner and announce: "Okay everybody, may I have your attention please? It's time for Lori's shot" then proceed to bend me over the table, my hair swaying over the stuffing as he does the deed, then take the ice off my ass and toss it back into his Sprite. It's called "prepping the relatives". If they can hold down their turkey through *that* escapade, they should have no problem digesting at future Thanksgivings should I sit next to them and breast-feed...topless... bottomless too if I feel like it.

"It's all in the wrist." Back in our innocent, pre-fertility issue days, that expression sparked to my husband only thoughts of putting a golf shot or shooting pool. Then we started our journey through fertility treatments. Soon he would realize that that simple phrase: "It's all in the wrist", was about to take on a much more ominous meaning.

Laughing *IS* Conceivable: Chapter Three

"It's All In The Wrist" aka **"I know what *you* just did"**

Women can endure anything. But ask a man to simply sit in a waiting room with a handful of strangers (in a moment you may consider "handful" to have been an unfortunate choice of words) who then pretend not to watch him accept a plastic cup and be ushered into a small room where they close the door behind him. Had this been a dentist's office, the cup could perhaps be for dentures. But this is a fertility clinic. Therefore, when the door opens again and he emerges, the audience looks stoic while thinking two things: The men think: "Oh no. I might be next" and *everyone* thinks:

"I know what YOU just did."

If women were called upon to do this task, we'd probably chat about it in the waiting room.

"This is the eighth time I've had to do this. I

hope it *takes* this time."

"You've done this *eight* times? You're my hero! I hope they take me soon. I have to pick up my daughter at gymnastics."

But men waiting to share some self-love with plasticware aren't big on eye contact or conversation. I've noticed that they are voracious readers though. Newspapers, books, matchbooks, the tags on the couch, nutritional facts on Snickers wrappers... Once I commented to my husband: "Why are these guys reading every magazine in the place? You don't have to choose one to bring in with you? I mean, they provide you with magazines once you get in there, don't they?" Needless to say, he doesn't sit next to me anymore. Although he himself commented once on a guy who was wearing a suit. We then discussed in depth the lack of practicality in this attire in terms of access and tidiness. We finally deduced that this

23

fellow likely had been in a meeting elsewhere and had not specifically put on a suit for this event at hand. (How many "palm puns" do I have in me?)

This Isn't Bridge. We Don't Need Four to Play.

I have a male friend who, upon exiting the donation room, discovered his in-laws in the waiting room awaiting his safe return---his mother-in-law's face a bright fuchsia. He was mortified. I set him straight. "Why should *you* be embarrassed? Serves her right. This is like her kid's prom. If she decides to chaperone, she gets what she gets."

My Husband's Respiratory Problems

Back when we first started with artificial insemination, we read over every piece of literature at they had given us. Seven hundred pages of my impending medications and shots and probings and scannings, and my husband was breathing quite normally. Two sentences about *him* "producing a sample in the doctor's office" and he spontaneously developed asthma. And for the next week, every time I turned over in bed, there he was in the dark, lying on his side with his one wide open eye staring back at me. It was like sleeping next to a goldfish that had quietly passed away in its bowl during the night. (I shouldn't talk about handling pressure. I could never be a professional tennis player. They only get ninety second bathroom breaks during the U.S. Open. My opponent, the officials, twenty-two thousand fans in the stands and eighteen million more at home staring at a half-empty court for a minute and a half, waiting for me to pee? Anyhoo...)

Every day, I was being checked to see exactly when I would be ready for insemination, so we never knew exactly when my husband's services would be called upon. Naturally, I can't relate to precisely what it's like for him, but I imagine it's a lot like working for a temp agency. I know when I was a temp, days were uncertain. I had to call in to the agency each morning, not knowing until that very moment if I was needed for work that day. Yeah, I'll bet that's what it's like for him. Next time he has to "give at the office", remind me to ease his mind with my temp theory.

And This Is The Torture Chamber Built In 1894

As the day got nearer for my husband to make his contribution, he was a wreck. They took us on a tour of the facility, which was a huge mistake. The tour nurse announced that the room where the guys are sent was "very nice and comfortable" as she flung the door open. The "honeymoon suite" consisted of a medical examination chair complete with that stripe of white crunchy-when-you-sit-on-it paper rolled down the middle and a dozen mangled magazines. Not quite the Playboy mansion. If that chamber didn't propel a man into impotency I don't know what would. I felt *my* testicles shrink. All in all, our tour of Hershey Park was considerably more successful.

At this point, my husband asked how I felt about sperm banks or if I thought that any of his friends were cute. Either option was fine with him. Then he came up with another strategy: Maybe he could do the lovin' at home and bring in the fruits of his "labor". The nurse said that was fine as long as we got the sample to them within ninety minutes of passion. No time for cuddling, naps, or cash transactions. I had images of *The Brady Bunch* episode in the amusement park when Dad's blueprints got lost and, once found, everyone took turns running with them to get them to the client before he got on a plane. (No Fedex then) I wondered if *The Lone Ranger* theme was going to play, as it did on that episode, as we were dodging taxis on the streets of Manhattan en route to the medical facility. At least I was pretty confident we weren't going to mistake my husband's sample for a Yogi Bear poster like dumb Jan did.

A Career Goal Dashed

With the pressure of having to produce in the doctor's office alleviated, my husband was in high spirits the morning of the deed. I, on the other hand, failed miserably as a porno princess (large breasts notwithstanding). Don't worry. I won't give details. There are none to give. He had made the mistake one day of telling me about "fluffing". Apparently there are women who work on porno productions whose sole purpose is to (by whatever means) get male actors ready, you know "ready" for the shoot. Those are the fluffers. Being the sex kitten temptress as well as loving and supportive wife that I am, that fateful morning I said to my husband in my most seductive and sultry voice:

"Hey, Baby, ready to get ffffluffed?"

He responded in his most loving and supportive voice:

"Could you just take a book and go outside?"

So whomever Debbie was doing in my DVD player, Lori was curled up with Agatha Christie on the cold, hard, cement steps.

My dad has a neighbor who likes to put her two cents into everybody's affairs. She can't accept the fact that my father is an older person who likes living alone, and is forever harping on him to hire someone to stay with him. Last week, Dad told me that he had a feeling that she wouldn't be bothering him about it anymore. With the barrage of unsolicited input I get these days on how to get pregnant and why I'm not pregnant, I was dying to know his secret.

"Wow Dad, how did you ever get her to leave you alone?" I asked, anxiously awaiting his sage advice.

"Simple." He said. "I told her to mind her own f----- business."

There are definitely some advantages to being eighty-five.

Laughing *IS* Conceivable: Chapter Four

"The Taming Of The Yentas"

No good ever comes out of lying. Unless you're going through what we're all going through and someone whom you don't want to know what you're going through asks you: "What are you going through?" Then lying brings an incredible sense of peace and well-being, accomplishment and self-satisfaction, joy and amusement.

I feel compelled to tell nobody but my husband the whole truth. With everyone else, I tell the truth, half-truths or just make up stories. So what if they're coworkers I see every day? So what if they're family? That doesn't automatically entitle them to any insider information. I've also been astounded to learn how many people who appear to be, shall we say, *limited* in both the common sense *and* book smarts departments, are experts in human reproduction in

31

general and mine in particular. I'm getting fertility advice from people who ask me every year what date Christmas comes out on and think Chicago is a state.

Who cares if my remarks make sense? Who cares if the story changes every time they ask me? If they ask personal questions, like the in-laws who chaperoned the sperm donation in the last chapter, they get what they get. This is a sample of me at the never-ending press conference:

"Excuse me, Mrs. Fox. Are you pregnant?"

Me: No. Ask any woman with big breasts. This is just how our shirts fit. Next question.

"Mrs. Fox, you've been married two years. Any plans for children?"

Me: We thought we'd have grandchildren first and see if we like it.

"Mrs. Fox, maybe you should have a baby NOW. Statistics show that the older you are the harder it is to conceive."

Me: Really? I hadn't heard that.

"Mrs. Fox, your sister-in-law has three children. Why don't you have any?"

Me: Those are actually *our* kids. We just keep them at her house.

"Mrs. Fox, why don't you take all of this money you're spending on medical procedures and go on vacation? Women *always* get pregnant on vacation."

Me: Yes I know. We're corporate sponsors of Club Med's annual baby shower.

"Mrs. Fox, ninety-eight percent of women get pregnant on their honeymoon. Didn't you and your husband have a honeymoon?"

Me: Yes at Disney World. We did it three times on Space Mountain and once in Cinderella's castle, but no luck.

"Mrs. Fox, all of your in-laws' neighbors' daughters-in-law have gotten pregnant. Why can't *you*?"

Me: I've heard it's good with pineapple.

"Mrs. Fox, is it possible that you and your husband

simply don't have enough sex?"

Me: It's possible. I'm not a morning person.

Whoever Miranda Was, She Understood Our Plight

I don't blame people for wanting to get into my follicles. Some people are truly concerned. Then again, some people are just yentas--- Nosy Nellies. In dealing with both categories, there are some strict rules I follow:

1) I have the right to make totally arbitrary, cryptic, and vague statements.

"When are you going to start a family?"

Acceptable responses: "We'll see.", "How about **you**?" "Good one!" "You never know." "You've got a point." "When God says so."

(The last one is the only one I've ever given as a sincere answer and the only one anyone has ever questioned me on. Go figure.)

2) **I have the right to share information with you today, but change my story or deny it altogether tomorrow.**

"In Vito what? What are you talking about? Isn't that 'Let the buyer beware' in Latin?"

3) **I have the right to stop giving information whenever I feel like it.**

"Didn't you go for a pregnancy test two weeks ago? How'd it turn out?!"

"We're working on it. Which reminds me: How'd your son do on his SATs?"

4) **I have the right to lie about anything and everything to do with this process.**

"They took seven hundred eggs out of me. Most women are only *born* with six hundred." Or:

"Oh, we gave up on all that months ago. We decided to buy a villa in Majorca instead."

5) **I have the right to let you or not let you discuss "my problem" amongst yourselves with no notice.**

In a get-together of some of my girlfriends, I

pulled this one while they were mid-whisper:

"I'm coming into the kitchen now! Everybody out of my uterus!"

At work, I see the little note pads dangling from the belt loops of the gossip hounds. They're just dying to know what I'm up to. I see them crouching under their desks to update their "Lori File":

Strange goings-on: Normally works at 6 a.m. but on CERTAIN days, arrives at 7:30 or 8:00. Last week it was Tuesday. Week before- Friday. Possibly having early morning affair with garbage man or newspaper delivery boy between houses.

Monday: Came in with Band-Aid on arm crease. (Not actual Band-Aid or even no-name bandage, but cotton ball stuck on with adhesive tape.) Same on Thursday. Possible heroin addict. Do junkies always shoot up in the exact same spot? Maybe she's just starting out. New boyfriend must be bad influence.

"Password is...... London Trip**"**

Then there's this London trip that I've shrouded in mystery. At last year's holiday party, I had the good fortune of winning a trip to London in the raffle. It's a barter deal my company has with the airline, so it's totally contingent upon when the airline says I can go. Welcome to the boxing match.

In this corner we have Eliza Doolittle Airlines: Won't offer trip during their busy season which includes but is not limited to: All holidays, rugby season, and periods of political unrest in Southeast Asia and Central Africa.

Then, in the opposite corner, we have Lori. Hormone taking, stomach injecting, mood swinging, weight gaining, pill popping, egg harvesting, Lori---with her own blackout days that keep her grounded, namely: Day two of every menstrual cycle for blood test and ultrasound. A few days later for same. A few days later for same. A few days later for same. Egg retrieval. Embryo transfer. Pregnancy test twelve days later. If positive: When will she be able to fly? If negative: Wash, rinse, repeat almost immediately. Ding! Ding!

The secretary who's handling this London business says I have to give at least a month's notice to take this trip. A month's notice? I live moment to moment. Cramp to cramp. Blood test to blood test. I'm waiting for the nurse to call to tell me if I have to go back in tomorrow or Saturday. You want me to tell you about the month after next? The secretary persists. Could I possibly take a month off from whatever it is I'm doing? Are you kidding me? And let my forty years, three months, two weeks and a day old eggs get thirty days---seven hundred and twenty hours--- older?

Management requests that I clarify why I can't

be more flexible regarding the "London Trip" and why I have to switch my work hours so often. "Personal business" just ain't cuttin' it for them anymore. They also know that I've bumped up my health insurance coverage. I state that I'm having a long-term "procedure" and close my lips. There are plenty of office yentas in management with their own branch of mumblings.

"What exactly is this 'procedure' she's having? She says she can't travel but she looks healthy. She runs to the doctor twice a week, but she also runs the two and a half miles home every day. Maybe she's a runner for a drug cartel: Taking phony prescriptions from doctors to pharmacists to hooded strangers on the street. Or maybe she's going to a cosmetic surgeon. Obviously didn't have her nose done. Clearly no breast reduction. She's not making them bigger is she? She wouldn't dare. Could be hormonal.

She did have that mood swing last month that we made her apologize to the entire accounting department for. Could be a sexual identity thing. Does seem to be growing an Adam's apple. May be why she's been wearing that woolen scarf all winter. Yep, every time the temperature's dropped into the teens, she's got that scarf on. That could be it."

I've always prided myself on being an honest person. Not one of those people at work who makes her way down three hallways and twelve cubicles to tell you how ugly your haircut looks because she's "just being honest". I have a good memory for numbers but a bad one for lies. So I never made lying one of my habits. But ever since I started going for baby help, I've been lying my tubes off. Not only to appease my doting public, but to amuse myself. I don't care if nobody believes me. I don't care if I'm inconsistent in what I tell them. It's like the song:

"Let's give them something to talk about. A little mystery to figure out." Bonnie Raitt was supposedly singing about love. Yeah right, Bonnie.

The other day I saw my medical file on the nurse's desk. Even upside down, I couldn't miss the big, flaming red capital "B" on the front of the chart. I have twenty-one letters in my entire name and not one of them is a "B". So what do you suppose that big, flaming red "B" that the receptionist, office assistant, accounts payable person, nurse, doctor, or some combination thereof wrote on my chart stands for? I wonder if, hidden somewhere in that office, there's a big, flaming red file cabinet containing all of the charts of all of their patients who have, like me, recently transformed into big, flaming red "B"s.

Laughing *IS* Conceivable: Chapter Five

"Be Nice To The Office Staff Or They'll Spit In Your Eggs"

When I call the doctors' office to ask a question or get test results, I have no problem asking for a specific nurse. Maybe I don't like Stephanie. She doesn't seem like she knows what she's talking about. No big deal. There are seventeen nurses. I'll ask for Diane or Laura or Julie.

Then there are the doctors. Well, I have eight of those. My impending conception is so important that I don't have one doctor. I have a team. Technically, I do have only one *main* doctor, but he may be in Bermuda or at his grandkids', or up to his elbows (literally) elsewhere when I'm ovulating. So I have that team of doctors scheduling their lives around my magnificent ovaries. If I don't care for one of their bedside manners, I can speak with someone else. BUT THERE IS ONLY ONE RECEPTIONIST!

43

She is the mistress of the entire office. She may be a Harvard graduate or a sixth grade drop-out. A lightning-speed thinker or have the common sense of a cotton ball. She may be Ms. Compassionate or Miss Nasty Pants. Either way, she alone can choose to grant or deny me telephonic access to all of the doctors, nurses, phlebotomists, anesthesiologists, billing people etc. etc. etc. If she stinks at her job or hates my voice and remembers it, I'm doomed. When I call, I always say "Good morning!!" like I'm hosting a morning show. If I forget and say it normally, I apologize for my rudeness and blame it on the hormones.

One office I went to, the girl was a dope. "Nasty" never sits well with me. But I can hang on a little longer with "stupid". When they're dumb AND rude I go berserk. It makes me want to go straight to the office, climb up on the reception desk, look straight down at them and yell: "You're a complete idiot! Now you're going to be snippy to me too?!" Luckily I've only actually had to do that twice...three times at most.

This dopy girl couldn't grasp the phone system. She was simply overwhelmed by the two lines. She could never decipher between which one was ringing and which one she had just put on hold. I don't know if it was a hand-eye coordination thing or what. She would just stare at the blinking light like she was getting a signal from Neptune or HBO. It would blink at her. She would blink back at it. It was truly something to behold in person. I was aching to reach over the desk and say "That's okay. I'll get it."

When she finally answered the phone, she did so very professionally: "Hello?" No name of the office. No "How may I help you?" There were two doctors in the office. She called them "Dr. P." and

"Dr. M.", I suspect, because "Pederson" and "Martin" were just too tough to master. At first I was sympathetic. I asked one of the nurses: "How's that new receptionist coming along? Any better?" She responded: "If you mean Jeannette, she's been here six years."

One day I called to get my blood test results. I was put on hold for about five minutes then dumped into the voice mail of the guy in charge of the sperm samples. When I called back, Jeannette apologized and transferred me directly to the actual guy, in person, who was in charge of the sperm samples. This poor guy did everything to try to help me but stick a needle in his vein and give me *his* blood results. Unfortunately, he was Jeannette's equal in maneuvering the phone system (ah, but how was *she* with sperm?) I finally just thanked him, hung up and tried spinning the Jeannette wheel again to see what I would get this time. It wasn't about test results anymore. It was strictly morbid curiosity.

This time the phone rang and rang. Finally, the doctor who ran the facility picked up. I said: "Dr. Martin, is that you? Where's Jeannette?" He answered, hope in his voice: "Maybe she quit."

How people like this stay employed, especially when so many qualified others are looking for work, is something I'm sure I'm much too unworldly to understand. But I feel sure it must involve "Dr. P." Clearly "Dr. M." doesn't find her quirks endearing.

Answering Services: Our Downfall As A Society

I don't necessarily believe that answering services will be our downfall as a society. But when I worked at one during college, a man expressed that very opinion when I picked up the phone at 8:45 one night instead of his accountant. Lately I've been empathizing.

One evening in the wee hours, maybe 10 p.m., I had a vital question to ask the nurse. I can't remember it now. Perhaps:

"Is it okay to shower during the eight days I'm injecting the Gonal F?" Or:

"I accidentally put one of the syringes in the refrigerator. Will it be cold when I use it?" Or:

"Last time I bought alcohol pads from CVS but my husband got these from Walgreen's. Are they okay to use or should I throw them out?"

Anyway, Nurse Diane was on call. We're buds. She loves me. So I called the answering service.

"Hi. I'd like you to page Diane when you have a moment."

"Diane's not on call. Only Dr. Bolger for emergencies."

"I'm positive Diane is on call. I'm a very

nervous person. She always lets me know when she's on call or leaving town."

"Only Dr. Bolger's on call for emergencies." (I won't say the fellow was totally disinterested, but until that moment, I never realized that you could actually hear someone looking at their watch.)

I remained focused. All at once, my years of dedication to *Columbo* and *Murder She Wrote* kicked in.

"Wait a moment, sir. Isn't Dr. Bolger's first name, Diane? Isn't it possible they told you that 'Diane' was on call and you just ASSUMED they meant Dr. Bolger?! Now **Nurse** Diane spells it D-I-A-N-E while I believe **Dr.** Dyan spells it D-Y-A-N like Dyan Cannon." (Why I thought this eight year old Thai boy would know who the hell Dyan Cannon is…)

Unmoved by my sleuthing skills, he refused to

veer from his "Only Dr. Bolger is on call for emergencies" mantra.

I really didn't want to page a doctor for a two second question that Nurse Diane could easily field. On the other hand, if the doc's all ya got…

Dr. Bolger returned my call about a half hour later. I thought she was going to reach out with her bare hands and do my egg retrieval right through the phone lines.

"*This* is what you called me for at 10 o'clock at night?! Why didn't you page Nurse Diane?!"

I recounted my ride on the "I'm positive Diane is on call" merry-go-round. I wanted to clear my name. But the more detailed I got, the more it sounded like a lie even to me. I should have just shut up and hung up. She needed time to not be a doctor and to figure out why I had the great "Diane or Dyan" debate when, lo and behold, her name was

Svetlana.

I also needed time: To figure out how to manipulate my follicles so that my retrieval and transfer would both take place on her day off.

They Conspire

Sometimes various branches of the office staff are in cahoots: Working in tandem to push me over the edge on which I already teeter. One afternoon, I still hadn't gotten that day's blood results. Granted, every day is the day I think the nurses are going to forget to call me with the evening's instructions. They never have. But on this day, it was 4:30 already. I called the office.

"Good Afternoon, doctors' office. Maria speaking."

"Hi, I'm calling for my blood results."

She doesn't tell me she's putting me on hold,

51

but either I'm on hold or Neil Diamond has recently joined the staff. I'm calm. I'm up for any *duet* that's not a prenatal vitamin. ♫"Money talks. But it can't sing and dance and won't cov-ver my shots. As long as you are here with me,... Hello? Hello? Maria? Are you here with me? Maria? Neil? Damn." I dial again.

"Good Afternoon, doctors' office."

"Good Afternoon, I just got disconnected. I was calling for my blood results."

"I'm so sorry. The office is closed. This is the answering service."

"I was just talking to them! I need my blood results! I have to know what to do tonight!"

"Please hold."

Entirely different person: "Good Morn... sh-t.*"*

She hangs up. I call back and get her again. She uses a fake high-pitched voice in an attempt to distance herself from her double faux pas--cursing and hanging up on a patient--triple if you count saying "Good Morning" at 4:36 p.m.-- but it's her alright.

"Good Afternoon, doctors' office. May I help you?"

"I was just explaining... I have to talk with someone in the office right away!"

"I'm sorry. The office is closed. This is the answering service. May I place you on hold?"

Obviously a rhetorical question because off she went. At least this one came back. She might curse and hang up on patients, but it's nice to know her "holds" are sincere.

"Thank you for waiting. I'm sorry. There's no one in the office at this time. May I take a message?"

"What did they all just rush out the door in the last thirty seconds? Look, if you can somehow just get me back to Maria, or at least 'Forever in Blue Jeans', Babe"...

I've dealt with mean-spirited administrative assistants who claim they never got your voice mails and, therefore, don't give doctors messages. I've dealt with incompetent billing people who've told me mid-cycle that I couldn't go through with the transfer because I hadn't paid a bill from the last cycle… that I'd already paid.

Look, it's not easy being women who for weeks, months, or years, are jumping through hoops labeled: "Hormone Altering" and "Life Altering". And it can't be easy dealing with us either. If you're not one of those extraordinaries on staff who can do a great job and also, somehow, smile through it, try this: While sitting at your office PC or laptop thinking up ways to spit in our eggs, log on to your local newspaper.com. Double click on "Classifieds". Scroll down to "Office Assistant-Dermatologist". Click. If you need a reference, call me.

I used to get so bored waiting in the waiting room for my thrice weekly blood siphoning appointment that once, to amuse myself, I whipped out a pair of cuticle scissors, hacked up a Ladies' Home Journal, and made a collage. The receptionist, who had mastered the art of registering patients without smiling, speaking, or looking up from her computer, called me. "Mrs. Fox?" I was so elated to hear her utter my name. It was like hearing Helen Keller say "water". I hurried over. She indicated my thumb and forefinger still attached to the cuticle scissors. "Mrs. Fox...Could you not do that anymore?" That's when my husband and I founded "The Waiting Room Games". Better than the Olympics: No commercial interruptions and always in your time zone.

Laughing IS Conceivable: Chapter Six

"Waiting Room Games"

I'm not a big magazine reader. And truthfully, I question some of the titles these doctors choose to offer in the waiting room: Parenting, American Baby… How about: Feeling Like Sh-t Monthly? The cover girl would be a stressed out, mood swinging woman in her bathrobe. I would probably flip through that one---one way or another. Let's face it. There are no appropriate magazines for this type of waiting room.

Men's Health- What guy's going to read that in a room full of women, and even worse...other men? Everyone will figure it's *him* not *her* that landed them here.

Travel + Leisure- Good. Let me read about places far away where I haven't been able to go for the past two years and won't be able to go for the next two years, because either I'll be doing this every month or I'll be having a baby. Either way, our funds will be so depleted, we'll be lucky if we can get to the nearest bus depot and back.

Family Circle- I have a family arc. We cannot naturally make a family circle. That's why we're here.

People- Nice. Let me see celebrities who get pregnant two weeks after their 3 million dollar dream wedding at a castle in Provence. Then the gestation period is somehow only a month, during which time they never weigh more than a hundred and five pounds, have heartburn, or throw up, but do look fabulous in a backless Valentino number coming down the red carpet. Then they have a beautiful healthy baby whom they stick with an idiotic name, hand off to a battery of nannies once the photographers have moved on, and never see again until the custody hearing. Or, even better, let me read about female celebrities who are having children at fifty-two, *naturally*.

Having exhausted the magazine options, and this office not providing any cool wooden puzzles or blocks like our dentist's office, my husband and I founded: **"The Waiting Room Games"**.

They are our answer (to a question nobody's ever likely to ask) to the Winter Olympics. Here's how they compare:

Winter Olympics
Held every four years at various locations around the globe. Participants must prepare mentally and physically, often for decades.

Waiting Room Games
Held every three days at our local doctor's office. Participants must show up and be bored.

Event #1: Who here is older than I am?

This event is not only fun, it also boosts my confidence. My husband never enters this event. He has no clue about, nor interest in, guessing women's ages behind their backs in front of their faces. While most women are in the room because they have (or at the very least suspect they *may* have) a problem conceiving, I'm jealous of the ones who look to be twenty-five. I figure that they have nearly twenty years to sort it all out, while I probably have up until and including Thursday. If I can only determine that a few of my co-waiting room waiters are *around* my age, then I can reassure myself that my doctor hasn't taken me on as a bet he made with the <u>New England Journal of Medicine</u>.

My cousin had a cat that was twenty-two years old. Every time she brought her to the vet, the whole staff would say: "Here comes that woman with that really old cat."

I know how that poor feline felt. I'm still relatively young: Ancient only by Hollywood and fertility standards. I often wonder if the office staff watches us getting off the elevator and mumbles: "Here comes that man with that really old wife." (Even though "that man" is actually nine days older than I am. But nobody seems to ever care about that.)

Event#2: "What Are YOU Doing Here?"

Every once in a while we see someone who cannot possibly be involved in IVF, but there they are! The place I go to inhabits the entire floor. When you get off the elevator, you can't be passing through on your way to anywhere else. One time we saw a nun in full nun garb. We tried for ten minutes to hallucinate the habit she was wearing into some sort of unfortunate wardrobe choice. We couldn't do it. Was she donating eggs? Is that allowed? We were stumped. It probably should have occurred to us that she was lending support to a patient. Of course nothing so plausible came to my mind until just now. My latest injections must be wearing off.

Also, every now and then, there will be a guy who seems to be in the waiting room by himself. Since the sperm sample is given right when the woman is about to be inseminated or the eggs are taken from her: Why is he by himself? Is he killing time until his movie starts? Did he see all of the ladies and have some warped notion that this office was a babe goldmine? Or did his new bride make him sit there so he can see where he could end up if he doesn't stop playing hockey goalie on the weekends? Oh, wait. Maybe he has male infertility issues that are being dealt with. Never occurred to me before. It's the nun thing all over again. Suddenly I'm V-8ing left and right. I really live in my own self-absorbed IVF hormone bubble, don't I?

Once we saw a woman who looked to be about six months pregnant in the waiting room. This place strictly tries to get you pregnant. No obstetrics. Did her dancing hormones make her confused and cause her to get off the elevator on the wrong floor? Or was she a shill for the facility? Maybe they pay a pregnant woman to sit in the waiting room to make us poor slobs think their success rate is higher than it is. (Nope. No light bulb coming on on this one. Didn't get it then. Still don't get it now.)

The people who really befuddle me are friends and relatives of those going through the procedures. I don't mean if a woman who would otherwise be alone, brings a buddy. I mean random aunts, uncles, and next door neighbors showing up. To these folks, I'm dying to yell out:

"I know what you're doing here. But WHAT are you doing here?! What do you live in a tiny town where high school soccer season is over? This isn't a spectator sport. If they were having a child in the usual way, would you set up bleachers outside their bedroom window?"

Once we saw an entire extended family nonchalantly lounging in the waiting room. They looked like they'd made a last minute decision to stop over on their way to IHOP.

"Mom, can I order a Rooty Tooty Fresh 'N Fruity with scrambled eggs?"

"That reminds me. Cousin Janis is having her egg retrieval today. Maybe we should swing by and see if she's in the mood for pancakes when the anesthesia wears off."

Event #3: IVF Veterans or Novices?

This event is a test of your ability to evaluate body language.

Couple #1: Husband and wife are sitting in adjacent chairs but as far away from each other as possible without her sitting on the armrest and him in a potted plant. He has brought all thirty sections of the Sunday <u>New York Times</u>.

To an untrained eye, it may appear that this man has had a busy week and wants to catch up on his reading. But those who have mastered this event know: These people are IVF veterans. Pros. Ringers. Deep down they love each other, but nobody cares about that right now.

Months ago, they made an unspoken pact: She agreed not to freak out, cry hysterically or wish him dead, if he would just shut up and stick his irritating face in a newspaper so she wouldn't have to look at it.

Since then, he has become the number one ranked Sudoku player in the world and memorized all of Marmaduke's vital and non-vital statistics. He could become a *Jeopardy!* champion or he may need a team of doctors for his failing eye sight, crick in his neck, and newsprint stains on his fingertips. No matter. During this process, a husband's got to do what a husband's got to do.

Couple#2: Both man and woman look intrigued by the magazine selection. They peruse several. Obviously new to this office. Probably novices altogether, since most offices have the same magazines. They're talking, holding hands, smiling nervously. This is like a date. Yep, they're newbies. They still like each other. That'll change. Neither has yet experienced the joy of her being curt to him all day every day, week after week, month after month, year after year. And he hasn't reached that moment when the only thing he has to look forward to in life is that fifteen seconds a night when he gets to stick her in the butt cheek with a long needle.

Couple#3: Husband and wife each hunt down a specific magazine. She announces that she needs the one with Jane Fonda on the cover. He grabs <u>Men's Fitness</u> and turns directly to page twenty-six. Clearly they've both been here before… and recently. They remember where they left off. (Either that or they are the most anal couple alive and asked the receptionist what periodicals the office subscribes to, then researched them on-line before showing up to their first appointment.)

Likely they have been involved with IUI/IVF for a few months. They know in which rack their favorite reading materials are usually buried, yet the excitement of free magazines has not yet worn off. She still appears genuinely grateful that he is accompanying her and has not yet graduated from: "It's so sweet of you to come to all of my appointments with me." to "There's nowhere else you could be?"

Event #4- Who's Doin' Whom?

For some reason, every time we're in the waiting room, there is an odd number of people. Is it a superstition of the office? "Sorry, we have an even number of people here. Someone has to go."

We always sit together. Others don't. In this event, we try to assess which woman is with which man. First we eavesdrop. Some couples never speak. Not to malign my own people, but I can't relate to this at all. Jews generally can't sit together for five minutes with nobody talking. Even if it's just to say: "You know that I'm not speaking to you, right? Did you hear me? Hel-lo?"

If two people sitting next to each other aren't talking, then we eavesdrop more intensely. Sometimes in this close, tense, setting, people are reluctant to chat but they will emit sounds: "Hm?" "Uh- Huh", "Na".

If we can still detect nothing, we move on to the superficial. Tall people are usually with tall people. Just like tan people are usually with tan people. Anyone knows that. That redheaded woman must be with that man. He definitely must have been a redhead before he lost all his hair. Everybody knows that redheads, like tall people and tan people, are clannish.

Then, over there---You can tell that that woman is shallow. She must be with that guy over there. You know she picked him so she'd have pretty babies. He may not even be her man. He may be "hired help". Just like those two over there must be together. They're about the same level of homely.

There is only one potential downside to the "Waiting Room Games". My husband and I are constantly comparing notes…aloud…and I'm usually speaking a whole lot louder than I think I am. This has led to another event in development tentatively called:

"We're *NOT* Talking About *YOU* and don't you have anything better to do than to spy on us spying on other people?!"

In this event, we'll confront the nosy Nellie (or Nelson) and ask them to figure out who **they** think we're talking about. It could be multiple choice. What do ya think?

I mentioned my little episode with the receptionist and my art project involving my cuticle scissors and their <u>Ladies' Home Journal</u>. I mentioned how said receptionist asked me, ever so politely, to "knock it off". I stopped short at mentioning how diplomatically I had responded. I calmly retreated back to my waiting room seat, pulled out a fistful of receipts from my tote bag, stomped back over to Sally Sunshine and said, shaking them in her face like I was a pom pom girl: "I'm sure somewhere in these eighteen thousand dollars, I paid for that magazine." Yeah, true, the receipts I waved before her were mostly from Target and added up to about five bucks worth of toothpaste and stockings. Still, I think I made my point.

Laughing IS Conceivable: Chapter Seven

"OOOOOOh Mr. Graaant"

I couldn't write an entire book without paying some small homage to *The Mary Tyler Moore Show*. Unfortunately, the "grant" I'm referring to here has nothing to do with Edward Asner, and everything to do with financial desperation.

I find expressions like "multitasking" to be idiotic. It's what people who text and drive say they're doing to feel important. I'll have to admit, it does sound better than: "I'm a moron risking everyone's life." But *we* are all the queens and kings of multitasking: Attempting to bear both children and a huge financial burden simultaneously. Isn't it great that in addition to worrying if you will ever have a baby, when it will happen, and whether both your body and your relationship will survive the process, you can tack on: "How in the world am I supposed to

71

pay for it all?"

Am I bitter? Yes. Do I hate rich people right now? Yes. Am I wrong for standing nose to nose with a stranger at Tiffany's and yelling in her face: "You know I could have every egg left in my body retrieved for the price of that necklace you're eyeing, you selfish tart!"? I don't think so.

SHE could go through the procedures over and over. SHE can try methods that won't even be available to the rest of us for thirty years. SHE can fly around the world to adopt a child! Okay, let me stop. For all I know, this is a penniless peasant coming in to shoplift. (Hey....No, I'd better not.)

Insurance is a wonderful thing. If mine covered anything, it would even be wonderfuller. I got into a confrontation with the Human Resources woman at my job. She took exception to the fact that I was telling this story to everyone I could find:

"By New York State law (the state in which I live and work), insurance is supposed to cover at least part of my 'procedure'. But because our headquarters is in another state that doesn't have this law, my company's insurance, by golly, isn't required to cover any of my costs after all. It's called the 'Lori loophole'".

I had gotten my information from the doctor's financial person. Well, when Ms. H.R. Pufnstuf at the home office got wind of my tale, she was incensed. She told me that the fact that the headquarters is elsewhere was not relevant. My "procedure", she explained, was not covered because of ERISA: The Federal Government's "Employee Retirement Income Security Act." Well, that made all the difference in the world, I can tell you. At the end of my "headquarters is in another state" story, my insurance company pays nothing and I'm screwed. On the other hand, at the end of her "ERISA" story, my insurance company pays nothing and I'm screwed. I felt so much better. I thanked her repeatedly for taking the time out of her busy day to make that phone call to set me straight.

In our quest for fetal funds, people have made some very creative suggestions, I must say. Even medical professionals brainstorm on my behalf. (Aren't you amused when doctors charge you an exorbitant sum, then suggest ways you can pay them faster? A chiropractor once told me that it would be cheaper if I paid six months of appointments up front. I'm about to ask if they'll take food stamps, and this loser makes me the generous offer of saving ten bucks a visit if I hand him six hundred dollars NOW.)

One doctor told us of patients who solicit everyone they know for funds: Their family, business associates, religious affiliations, and general community at large. What would be a clever ad to put in the penny saver?

"Like the Fox family? Want to help make more of them?" (It would have been cleverer to say: "Want to add to our skulk?", but I didn't even know that was what you called a group of foxes until I just looked it up.)

Let's hold a bake sale! Or maybe a car wash! I even know the sign I would hold up: "Car Washing for Sperm Washing"

I suppose my point is: The whole community spirit thought is a beautiful one if you don't mind everyone knowing your business. Talk about pressure. Wouldn't you look forward to the corner grocer tapping you on the shoulder while your head's in the milk refrigerator?: "Are we pregnant yet?"

Wouldn't you love your boss saying: "I sank five grand into this project. When am I going to see some results?"

I envision us finally having a baby and ending up in a custody hearing with some yokel: "Hey, I've invested in that kid. He's ten percent mine! I should get him every other Easter!" Still, even though it's not for me, I wouldn't dare judge anyone who chooses the option of soliciting their friends, relatives, or community. Ya gotta do what ya gotta do.

Then, one doctor made a suggestion that to me was outrageous. I don't hold it against him. He knew it was outrageous, but wanted us to know it was an option, albeit an outrageous one. I think he even prefaced the idea with: "I know this sounds outrageous…"

He told me that there was a possible way around the insurance debacle: Another "Lori loophole" (this one in my favor.) See, if I had some sort of surgery, something inserted through my belly button to see if I had endometriosis, then it was possible that the insurance would then pay for the surgery and ANY procedures following (i.e. IVF wink wink). Of course, he had no belief whatsoever that I had endometriosis and told me that it wouldn't matter if I did because IVF bypasses that problem anyway. To sum it up: It was about having a surgical procedure solely to appease (or "rip-off" if you prefer) the insurance company. I had managed to successfully duck surgery my entire life. I wasn't about to start with a medically unnecessary one. I told him: "Thanks for the suggestion. I would rather collect twenty thousand dollars in Coke cans." (They give you five cents for each one in New York.)

Here are some *real* ideas that we've come up with on our own or stolen from others:

1) **The price of all services is like the admission fee at the Metropolitan Museum of Art: Only a suggestion.**

We treat the whole thing like a reverse auction: They say: "It's five thousand dollars". We say: "Do I hear *three* thousand?" You'd be surprised how many people get deals this way. It may feel uncomfortable at first, but pride don't pay the progesterone. Once I went in only for blood tests. The bill for that day was two hundred dollars. I asked the cashier: "Don't you sell anything in this joint for fewer than three digits?"

2) **See if your doctor has deals.**

Fertility places are so popular nowadays we'll probably start getting circulars in the mail: "Look Honey, Dr. Benson is having a 'freeze the second one free' sale!" Seriously, a lot of places will offer you a discount on the second go-round of treatment--even bigger discounts if you're under thirty-five. (They told *me*: "Are you kidding Granny? Loved you on *The Beverly Hillbillies* though.")

3) **Save every single pharmaceutical-sounding receipt for the insurance company.**

I lump together receipts for Follistim and Gonal F with ones for tampons, Q-tips and vitamins. If the ink's run out on the cash register tape, I still submit the half-blank receipt. Sure, I know there's probably a guy working at the insurance company who dumps my envelopeful on his desk, sifts through the pile and mumbles: "What the f… is this supposed to be?"

And right, Ms. HR Pufnstuf at my company *did* say that our insurance covers nothing. Yet every once in a while, I get a check in the mail. I never wait to find out if it's a mistake. I leave the mailbox door flung open, jump in the car, and hurry to the bank. Months later, I read my insurance statement and have no idea what they're talking about. I don't mind. As long as I can give the check to the teller at the drive-up window and get a receipt with my lollipop, I'm good.

4) **Here's something I haven't tried yet, but have heard good things about**:

Doctors who don't normally take your insurance agreeing to a special assignment with your insurance carrier. I can see me trying to finagle that. (What *can't* I see me doing at this point?)

"Okay, Dr. Smith. I hear you don't take my insurance. How about I take you and my Aunt Aetna out to lunch tomorrow? Meet me at the drive-thru at noon. I'll be in the red Corolla."

"Welcome to Wendy's. May I take your order?"
"Yeah, you see the guy behind me in the gray Jaguar and the group behind him in the corporate jet?! They're with me! Give them whatever they want! No, nothing for me thank you! I have just enough to cover the Jag and the jet! Sorry I'm yelling! My window hasn't worked since 2003!"

Actually I think these special assignment agreements are all done via mail and fax--- no fast-food bribe required.

5) **Don't forget about your Flexible Spending Account.**

My insurance carrier may refuse to pay for anything and everything (Have I mentioned that before?), but I'm FSAing my way through the year. You know about FSA/Flexible Spending Account/Follistim Savings Account, right?

I put as many pre-taxed dollars on it at the beginning of the year as I can afford without us having to eat dinner at a different nurse's house every night. Last year I could only swing five hundred dollars. It was still worth it. I used it for co-pays, deductibles, whatever…and they took only nineteen dollars and seventy-three cents out of my check every two weeks. I was so anxious that I wouldn't use it up before it expired at the end of the year. I didn't want to be like Cinderella running to a fertility pharmacy on New Year's Eve. Turns out there really was no cause for panic. I bankrupted the account circa January 20th.

6) **Here's where the "grant" thing I mentioned like eleven pages ago comes in.**

Get on your computer and research, research, research. You may be pleasantly surprised to find places: Government agencies, private agencies, charities… that might offer assistance for fertility treatments. I sat and cried in a doctor's office while I enumerated our financial woes. He never once mentioned that since 2004 and through at least the writing of this book, New York State has had a grant program in place. (NYS Infertility Demonstration Program) Did he not know about it? Or did he not want to know about it because he didn't participate in it? I applied and got it. It's amazing. Unfortunately, I hear it's also a one-of-a-kind program. Contact your state health department. See if they offer anything at all: Even suggestions where else to hunt. Familiarize yourself with the insurance laws for your state. Some require a portion of IVF to be covered. Some don't, but require other expenses surrounding infertility to be covered. Check Resolve.org for info and INCIID.org (pronounced "inside") for info and scholarships. Be creative. Be open. Be flexible. I mean don't go to Marco the Mechanic for your next egg retrieval just to save cash and get a free lube job... You're a smart cookie, you know what I mean.

.

I'm not going to go as far as to say that you ever lose sight of your goal of having a baby while going through all of these treatments. It's just that, for me, I got so caught up in my infertility bubble. For the better part of forty years, my life's routine had been: Get up in the morning, brush my teeth, get dressed, go to work. Suddenly, it had been drastically altered to months and months of: Get up, etc. etc., get on the train, walk five blocks to the fertility clinic, take the elevator to the third floor, sign in at the desk, give blood, go to work, wait for the phone call from the nurse, do the nightly needle ritual. I think my mind sort of tuned itself out---desensitized itself---to all of the steps of fertility treatments so I could somehow continue with the rest of my life while doing what I had to, to try to conceive. I think my mind put all of that stuff into its own little compartment labeled "Baby Making" so that I could still function: Hold a job, have friends, drive a car without the enormity of it all suffocating my brain. I hadn't realized, of course, that this was happening at the time. Not until that one day at the end of December, when I was at work and the nurse called me on my cell phone. I saw the extremely familiar number come up as I fumbled to get the phone out of my pocketbook under my desk. As I answered it with my hands starting to dampen and shake, I jogged through a sea of cubicles, down two hallways, through the kitchen, and out onto a roof deck to try to find some privacy.

"You're pregnant." She said.

I hung up and mumbled to myself.

"That's impossible. How could this have happened?" And for about twelve seconds, I really was serious.

Chapter Eight/Afterword

"Will the Months and Months of Madness (N)Ever End?"

The short answer is: "Absolutely". I wanted to sub-title this chapter/afterword something like: "My Wind-Up" or "My Final Fertility Chapter" but I didn't want you to see it in the Table of Contents and skip to the end of the book just to see how my travels turned out. That's what I would have done.

I certainly hope you have enjoyed this little book and found some comfort hidden among the wise-ass remarks. While I do tend to lean a little toward exaggeration and a lot toward sarcasm, almost all of the anecdotes truly happened as I reported them to you. Now to fill in any blanks:

In 2002, I was a single woman---never been married---no kids---living like a lot of single women in the boroughs of New York City: Up four elevatorless flights of stairs in a three room apartment, with no laundry in the building, windows that wouldn't stay open, others that wouldn't stay shut, heat that I couldn't control, and feeling pretty damn smug because I was paying less than a grand a month for the privilege.

My friendly neighborhood gynecologist was a man in his sixties. His wife/receptionist used to joke how I was going to be the oldest woman to ever have a baby and he was going to be the oldest doctor to ever deliver one. Hilarious. I was about thirty-five when I started going to him. (If he'd been a doctor in Manhattan, nobody would have blinked an eye at me. Due to the overwhelming demand there, some ob/gyns have intentionally geared their practices toward women over thirty-five.)

This doctor and I had the same dialogue at every yearly visit. He would say:

"You shouldn't be waiting this long to have a

baby." Then I would say:

"I don't even have a boyfriend."

Then he would brandish a photo of his three charming grown boys and boast:

"Sorry, mine are all taken."

At the third annual go-round, I chose to end the scene a little differently. After his stale: "Sorry, mine are all taken" line, I retorted, throwing a glance toward the photo:

"So? Who wanted them?" And found a different doctor.

Of course I knew his basic advice was on target all along: I shouldn't have been waiting so long to have a baby. I once read an inane article called something inane like: "Oops, I forgot to have a baby" about women who get so wrapped up in being a force in the business world that life just gets past them and they wake up one morning at forty and say: "Oh, I'd better get on that baby project." I'm sorry. That sounds absurd to me. We're not morons. Are there really women in this day and age who don't know about the whole biological clock thing? Is there any woman flirting with thirty-five or beyond who wants to have children who's not starting to freak out just a little? But what choice did I have?

I had some fleeting nutty thoughts. I have a gay pal from college who's in a great relationship. Maybe he could father my child? Then, I have another gay friend who wanted to have a baby. But his family is a mess: He, as well as everyone in every generation as far back as I know-- on both sides of his family-- is an alcoholic. I mightily applaud all of them who are in recovery, but there still was no way I was taking a plunge into that gene pool. If I had fallen in love with a man in that family, I would have had to make that tough decision. But that wasn't the case. I finally had a long talk with myself and realized that I didn't just want to have a baby. I wanted a romance...a relationship...a marriage...and then, if possible...a family.

So, there I was, in the early 2000s, pushing thirty-nine (as far away as I could) with no personal prospects. It was December and I hadn't had one date that entire year, yet it was a vast improvement over the year before when I'd had a handful. One lived with his sister in a two room basement apartment. Our date was spent watching Italian soccer on their TV... with her... and their cousin. (I love sports but not TV soccer.) Another guy was my one and only foray into on-line dating. Somewhere between my desktop and the restaurant, he lost six inches in height. Or am I miscalculating? You tell me. If I'm 5'3" (more in my dreams than in the doctor's office) and wearing two inch heels, and a man is 5'11", when we're standing side by side, should I be able to see the top of his head? His height white lie notwithstanding, any warmth and personality he had on the computer had evaporated into cyberspace. He spent the whole dinner telling me what a great catch his family thought he was and how they just couldn't understand why he was still single. I wanted to call them all on speaker phone and say: "Here. Listen to *this*." Instead I spent an hour and eighteen minutes singing the scores to *Rent* and *Annie Get Your Gun* in my head to keep from snoozing in my salmon which, in my opinion, was the only great catch at that table. (Did I just insult myself?)

Then it happened. I met my future husband in the way most do: At a gay Hanukkah party. I told you I have a lot of gay friends. They ran this social event. They wanted a big turn out, so everyone: Gay/straight, male/female, married/single was invited. And I couldn't get out of it. I was thrilled to have to schlep out on a below zero December night to slap down twenty bucks for the honor of dancing with a gaggle of gay men. I didn't brush my hair. I didn't change out of my sweats and T-shirt. I definitely didn't bother with make-up. I may not have even put on a bra. (And believe me, at 34D, I'm not one of those women who asks her girlfriends: "I don't really need one, do I?")

So here I am, going to a party in my "I'll just run out and get the mail" attire. I'm there about an hour, making the most of it by acting stupid and dancing some Israeli folk dancing/mashed potato hybrid in a circle with some of my straight women friends who had also gotten roped into attending. Two cute guys walked in the door. (Force of a twenty year habit, I was checkin' 'em out.) A few minutes later, one of the event organizers made his way over to our loop of losers.

"There's a guy over there who wants to dance with a woman" he said.

I was game. Did I have any dignity at all at this point? On my way over, I wondered what kind of a lame gay guy this was who had a sudden epiphany about dancing with a female. Maybe it was on a dare. Turns out he grew up with this guy who had just "come out" and who wasn't comfortable socializing yet. My guy was being a good Samaritan and attending the party so his friend wouldn't have to go it alone. Well, that was his story anyway. I still believe it. That summer we got engaged. The wedding was in the fall.

I don't believe that long engagements are as important when you're older. I always say that searching for a mate is like clothes shopping. When you're twenty, you pull everything off the rack and try everything on. Some you leave in the dressing room. Some you bring home and return later, ultimately realizing that the fit wasn't quite right. When you're thirty-five, you should be able to just open the door, poke your head inside the store, say: "Nope. Nothing here for me" and keep on your merry way down the sidewalk.

But don't think the fertility issue didn't play a part in our decision making. We both wanted a child. Our parents weren't getting any younger and neither were we. My husband is exactly nine days older than I. By the time we got married, we were both thirty-nine and a half. I personally don't think that I would have had any trouble conceiving if I had tried younger. But who knows?

We started trying the day we got married. For a year, I followed ovulation dates and did home pregnancy tests with no success. My forty-first birthday was about a block and a half away when we finally dragged our heels, kicking and screaming, into a fertility joint. They were shocked that my hormone levels were still as high as they were. I tried artificial insemination. I have never heard of anyone getting pregnant by IUI. If you have, please let me know. Maybe I'm traveling in the wrong circles.

That first lab-done pregnancy test result was one of the most devastating. Your hopes are so high. You really don't know what you're dealing with yet. That was the day I found out that something I had always believed to be true was a total lie: You can indeed be "a little pregnant". The result was a low-positive. What the hell does that mean? I found out what that meant soon enough. It meant that something fertilized but wasn't growing... so forget about it...and try again.

I had three unsuccessful shots at IUI. The

fourth one was done at a different facility. I told them that, judging by my previous go-rounds, my follicles (the sac in which the egg grows and matures) seem to grow a lot on their own at the end and that maybe I didn't need a final dose before the insemination. They decided that they knew better and told me to take one more dose. When I went in for my final IUI attempt, my levels were so high that it had to be canceled. On to IVF (in vitro fertilization).

The orientation was very disorienting… and depressing. We sat around with a group of other IVF hopefuls and perused stacks of literature while a nurse guided us through. What I gleaned from all of the statistics and charts was that at my age, (now forty-one) I had a better chance of a twin-engine plane landing in my driveway than I did of ever getting pregnant. And I didn't have a driveway… so I was really depressed. B'dum bum.

We had already come this far, so we decided to press on. In your average egg retrieval for any woman of any age, I was told, usually six to eight eggs are taken out. They grabbed twenty-one out of me. A few days later, sixteen of my eggs had fertilized nicely. They graded my eggs/embryos in order of how they assessed their quality. All got A's and B's. I went for the deed to be done.

They told me as I dressed for the procedure that due to my age, they were going to implant the four top contenders if it was okay with us. Of course we agreed. I mean, is this the best time for a couple to be making this decision? I mean, who was I to argue? I had on paper booties for chrissakes.

None of them took. We had been informed at the disorientation that frozen embryos had a much lower success rate than the fresh, but hey, at this point we were ready to sprinkle a few in the backyard and see what came up in the spring.

They defrosted my potentially future family: The next best four. Three of them still looked great. A female doctor implanted them. I say "female" doctor because not long after this procedure, another long-believed myth was disproved: A woman *can indeed* get another woman pregnant. Those three thawed out embryos are now our family and affectionately known as Triplets A, B, and C. (Will they grow up and resent us for not giving them actual names? Only time will tell.)

This entire book, with the exception of this final chapter, was written while I was going through the uncertainty of infertility. I thought it vital to be writing to you from the trenches. I didn't want to sound disingenuous by regaling my struggles when I already knew that the outcome was eventually good. Once I had the children, I felt that I would be gypping you if I didn't tell you the wind-up of my fertility saga, now that it had one. As hellish as it all was, I like to believe that I went through it then, so that in some small way, I could help you- yes, *you*- go through it now.

It's extremely important to me that you somehow keep your sense of humor during this time. Obviously the issue couldn't be more serious, but how ridiculous are some of the steps and comments and advice, and yes: How ridiculous are some of the *people* you have to deal with? I couldn't have handled it without constantly conducting a diligent search for the lighter side of it all. I was so wound up, so stressed out. I either had to laugh or go totally mad. I mean, I could have let myself freak out if this whole thing had taken a week or two, but I couldn't live month after month or year after year like that…and neither can you.

Getting pregnant, I found out, was only battle number one. Being pregnant with triplets came with its own litany of negative statistics. At this point, I was choking on pie charts. At my age, I should never have found a good husband. I should never have had twenty-one eggs yanked from my loins. Frozen embryos shouldn't have grown into healthy (albeit frequently trying) children. During the pregnancy, at least one of my vital organs should have exploded. I should have been on bed rest. I should have had several hospital stays along the way. The point is: I could have panic attacked my way through it all and NONE OF IT EVER HAPPENED.

And maybe...just maybe...none of it ever happened *because* I didn't panic attack my way through it all. I mean, is a stressed out, freaked out body the place most conducive to conceiving a child or growing a healthy one? For that matter, will a stressed out, freaked out parent be the best one to raise the child? This is why I think that it is imperative to listen intently to all of the medical advice, but also to try hard to keep some perspective- some sense of humor amidst all the insanity. Laugh now. Find the peace now. Take everyone with a grain of salt. Please don't flip out over every thoughtless, half-assed remark a relative makes or because the woman down the block had a bad experience. If you can't walk away altogether, do all you can to not overreact, keep a smile on your face, and most important: Learn the lyrics to a lot of show tunes.

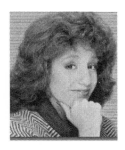

About the Author

Lori Shandle-Fox is a humor writer and former stand-up comic. Her humor and non-humor bits and pieces have appeared in: <u>The Washington Post</u>, <u>The Philadelphia Inquirer</u>, <u>Newsday</u>, and <u>Reader's Digest</u>, and on NPR and GrokNation.com. Her Laughing IS Conceivable book and blog series are designed to de-stress people from life's anxieties big and small- all stressful times that she herself has experienced.

Lori is a native New Yorker currently living in North Carolina. She and her husband Lloyd remain committed fans of their New York sports teams. (For better or worse, till death do they part.)

Laughing IS Conceivable... And Humor Heals

What the Experts are Saying about
<u>Laughing *IS* Conceivable</u>

"Laughing IS Conceivable is like a breath of fresh air and will be a welcome antidote to individuals and couples who are searching for a new way to relieve the stress of their infertility."

Alice D. Domar, PhD
Executive Director- Domar Center for Mind/Body Health
Director of Mind/Body Services at Boston IVF
Author, <u>Conquering Infertility</u>

"...Laughing IS Conceivable is a must read for all patients, partners and family members going through this process. Lori's humorous look at the patient, as well as the medical side of this treatment journey is refreshing and needed."

Richard P. Marrs, MD
Founder and Managing Partner, California Fertility Partners- Los Angeles, CA
Author: <u>Dr. Richard Marrs Fertility Book</u>

"When you smile, life smiles with you, and in this book, Lori Shandle-Fox shares...how humor uplifts us in the most challenging of times. Infertility is hard, yet when you add a spark of humor to the journey, the light shines and improves the experience and, I

believe, the outcome. Thanks to Lori for sharing many laughs."

Robert J. Kiltz, MD, FACOG
Owner & Director CNY Fertility Centers,
CNY Healing Arts
Author: The Fertile Secret, Guide to Living a Fertile Life

"Having cared for infertility patients for over 30 years, I loved this book. Lori writes: 'How ridiculous are some of the people you have to deal with.' Amen. Lori has a wonderfully entertaining and light-hearted way of discussing a serious, sensitive, and frustrating subject..."

Laurence A. Jacobs MD, FACOG
Partner- Fertility Centers of Illinois
Integramed Practice

"Hilarious! I would highly recommend Laughing IS Conceivable to anyone who needs a good laugh as they go through infertility treatments."

Eve Feinberg, MD
Assistant Professor, Northwestern School of Medicine
Medical Director, Northwestern Fertility and Reproductive Medicine- Evanston, IL

"...Lori Shandle-Fox is an insider. Not preaching at us about how we should feel, instead shifting the lens

so we can appreciate the laughable about the trials and tribulations of infertility treatments...And yeah, you bet I ended up laughing so hard I cried a little... I wish that every Reproductive Endocrinologist would include Lori's book as their treatment protocol. Write a prescription for it!

Lisa Rosenthal
Patient Advocate
Reproductive Medicine Associates of Connecticut
RESOLVE New England Board Member

"Laughing IS Conceivable offers the right dose of medicine for coping with infertility- humor. Lori's journey offers tremendous insight and comfort in a shared experience of infertility... This book is a must read for anyone experiencing infertility who embraces the notion that laughter is the best medicine."

Andrea Mechanick Braverman, PhD
Clinical Associate Professor of Psychiatry
Thomas Jefferson University, Jefferson Medical College, University of Pennsylvania

"Lori Shandle-Fox's book...reveals some of our hidden thoughts, fantasies and frustrations, reducing the pain and joining us with countless other women suffering infertility, while bringing fun into our life for a time. Read it, you will feel better".

Jean Benward, Psychotherapist
San Ramon, CA

"Hilarious descriptions of the sometimes absurd situations that fertility patients find themselves in. ...My guess is that many a patient, physician, receptionist, and nurse will be able to see (and laugh at) a bit of herself in this book."

Annette Lee, MD
Medical Director of IVF Program
Toll Center for Reproductive Sciences
Abingdon Reproductive Medicine
Eastern Pennsylvania

"Lori Shandle-Fox has considerable experience in making people laugh, and has done so again at her own expense...I smiled and related to her personal battles as I believe will most, if not all couples experiencing this emotionally and financially draining circumstance".

Bobby Webster MD
Medical/Practice Director
A Woman's Center for Reproductive Medicine
Baton Rouge, LA

"When people struggle to conceive, stress levels run high enough to put them at risk for serious mental health issues such as depression and anxiety

disorders. This wonderful book... is highly recommended for anyone struggling to conceive and their friends, family, and support network."

Serena H. Chen, MD
Director of Reproductive Medicine
St. Barnabas Medical Center, New Jersey

"IVF is probably the most emotional, stressful, mood swinging, (I could go on) period in an infertility patient's life.... I LOVE, LOVE, LOVE this book...and recommend it to all my patients."

Suzanne Degelos, PhD
Lab Director
The Center for Reproductive Medicine
Mobile, AL

"You know a book about a serious topic like infertility is accomplishing the mission of lightening the burden when you're on chapter 3 and realize that your face has been frozen in a smile for 25 pages. What a talent - to make the un-funny, funny. "

Helen Adrienne, LCSW, BCD
Psychotherapist, Clinical Hypnotherapist,
Practitioner of Mind/Body Therapy
New York, NY
Author: On Fertile Ground: Healing Infertility

*"When I am taking care of my patients, I try to be kind and friendly and, at times, funny. Lori Shandle-Fox's book is fantastic and funny and so true. All patients who are about to embark on treatment should read it as it would make them realize that they are not alone in their feelings: Keep your eye on your goal, laugh at times and let your fertility team do their magic to help you become pregnant. Thank you, Lori, for writing such a funny, true and important book which even made **me** laugh. Truly love it."*

Spencer S. Richlin, M.D.
Partner and Surgical Director
Reproductive Medicine Associates of Connecticut